Natural and Prescribed Treatments for Adrenal Fatigue

Choosing the Best Treatment for Exhausted Adrenals

By: James M. Lowrance   © 2010

TABLE OF CONTENTS:

INTRODUCTION:

This book is compiled from articles I wrote on the subject of adrenal fatigue between the years 2005 and 2009 that contain information on conditions commonly related to the syndrome, with emphasis on treatments that are available, of both the prescribed and natural types. Included in the information is discussion on the most suspected causes for diminished adrenal gland function, resulting in symptoms. Within these discussions, I point out both the successes and failures reported by medical research groups, who have tested the efficacy of cortisol steroid hormone treatments for patients with sub-clinical forms of adrenal insufficiency. I also discuss the positive results that other adrenal fatigue patients experience with alternative and natural self-treatments.

The importance for recognition by the medical community for adrenal fatigue syndromes is also an included aspect within the chapters that follow and I dedicate most of the final chapter in this book, to the subject of conventional-medical versus alternative-natural treatments, pointing out the reality that both can be positive or negative, depending on each case they are administered for.

This latter aspect is not included, to confuse the reader but to simply point out that patient-individuality comes into play, as well as trial and error, when superior treatments are being sought for individuals with adrenal fatigue syndromes.

The point is hopefully conveyed adequately, that options for treatments are not restricted to one type but that some adrenal fatigue patients can respond favorably to more that one type treatment or in some cases, to a combination of them. Through patient self-education and pro activeness, optimal treatment can be found but understanding the causes of adrenal fatigue for an individual and knowing whether or not there are co morbid conditions present (related, coexisting ones) can help with the determination for treatment options. With thyroid disease being common in adrenal fatigue sufferers, I also dedicate a portion of the information that follows, to the relationship of thyroid to adrenal function.

It is my sincere hope that readers will benefit from the information contained within the chapters of this book.
-*Jim Lowrance*

CHAPTER 1:

Adrenal Fatigue by Any Other Name

Many Doctors pronounce patients "normal" in regard to their adrenal function when they pass the tests they feel are the only ones needed to diagnose low adrenal function. These will often be the "ACTH Stimulation test" and/or a snapshot blood cortisol reading (the major adrenal stress hormone). The problem is that adrenal fatigue is a condition of disrupted "cortisol rhythm" and is not necessarily due to cortisol being low all of the time or because the adrenals can't be stimulated. Adrenal fatigue is not usually found until a multi-reading test is performed to gauge a patient's readings of cortisol, over a 24 hour period. Even a test that takes two readings -- one at morning upon waking when cortisol levels are supposed to be highest and one at midnight when levels are supposed to be lowest can help to give a cortisol average, rather than just a single snapshot level.

What really convinced me years ago, that mild adrenal dysfunction does exist and has been proven in medical research, are those medical research articles published in regard to syndromes like CFS (Chronic Fatigue Syndrome).

His includes information published on Fibromyalgia and PTSD (Post Traumatic Stress disorder) as well. These articles clearly state that people with these type syndromes often suffer low cortisol levels and they have also found a strong association of these syndromes to chronic stress, of either the prolonged type or the type caused by sudden traumatic events.

Here are example research article quotes:

"Several years ago, Dr. Straus and his colleagues found that CFS patients had slightly lower levels of circulating cortisol, the major glucose-regulating stress hormone, than did healthy individuals. Doctors have long believed that even subtle deficiencies in cortisol can result in lethargy and fatigue." (http://www.niaid.nih.gov/news/newsreleases/1998/pages/cfs.aspx)

"Both fibromyalgia and CFS are often viewed as being stress-response related, and abnormalities of the HPA axis have been found in both disorders.
...
In our study, morning cortisol levels were lower in women with CFS than in healthy controls.

Some studies of the HPA axis in CFS show a mild hypocortisolism of central origin, in contrast to hypercortisolism of major depression.

...

Cortisol levels peak in early morning and need to be collected before patients rise in the morning; and determining single levels of hormones that are secreted in a pulsatile fashion may not be representative of normal functioning."
(http://www.medscape.com/ -- "Cortisol and Hypothalamic-Pituitary-Gonadal Axis Hormones" © 2004 BioMed Central, Ltd. verbatim copying and redistribution permitted)

"Post-traumatic stress disorder is often associated with low production of cortisol."
(http://psychiatry.jwatch.org/cgi/content/full/2007 /1210/1)

While research articles do not use the term "adrenal fatigue", this is exactly what is being described by them. They will instead use terms such as "mild adrenal insufficiency", "blunted HPA axis", "hypocortisolism" or simply "low cortisol".

These type research articles are out there in significant numbers, so doctors who still do not believe that sub-clinical adrenal insufficiency conditions exists, need to take a look at a few of these published studies.

Adrenal fatigue by whatever other name they wish to call it does exist and is found in a variety of stress-related syndromes.

CHAPTER 2:

Adrenal Fatigue and Thyroid Patients

A lot of patients with thyroid disease also have some co-existing adrenal fatigue.

Add to thyroid disease, something like a traumatic or very stressful even and you can really suffer from adrenal fatigue. Your circadian rhythms are off with this condition and is why sleep patterns may also become disrupted. Your "cortisol" and "DHEA" (the two major adrenal hormones) will have their peaks, at the wrong times, such as at sleep time and your normal drop in these hormones also happens at the wrong time, like during the day, when you most need the peak-energy. Adrenal fatigue that continues for a long period of time (chronic) may then become "adrenal exhaustion" and this is the point at which you no longer experience those needed peak levels at all.

I have had adrenal fatigue for several years, as a feature of Chronic Fatigue Syndrome and co morbid to my autoimmune thyroid disease (Hashimoto's thyroiditis) and I have also experienced adrenal exhaustion.

Mine turned into adrenal exhaustion, after experiencing the onset of hypothyroidism and after having gone through a period of severe, prolonged stress.

Mine did not improve when I first began thyroid hormone replacement but actually worsened for a time. After several months on the correct thyroid dose, I finally saw some improvement in thyroid and adrenal symptoms. At times of extra stress and extended periods of hard physical activity, I've taken some adrenal support supplements, that I learned about when first researching about adrenal fatigue and these have helped a great deal. These include multi "B" vitamins, especially B-12, in sublingual form (liquid) and vitamin C, magnesium, selenium, zinc, DHEA 25mg (over-the-counter adrenal hormone) and sometimes but less-often, an Adrenal Cortex Extract (processed beef adrenal glands in pill form).

These always help me a great deal during flares of adrenal fatigue but I don't take the ones containing actual trace amounts of adrenal hormone (cortisol), as a permanent regimen. However, as safe as they are purported to be at the recommended doses, it likely would not hurt for me to do so if I felt it was necessary at some point.

I considered taking a cortisol drug called "Cortef" (natural adrenal steroid) and I had a Dr. willing to treat me with it but I was slightly wary of steroids, even at low doses and I still am. I have however, read many reputable medical resources stating that Cortef is safe as physiological doses (25mg and less), to supplement a person's low cortisol levels from adrenal exhaustion but the hormone drug can cause "adrenal suppression", if administered in full replacement doses (above 25mg -- but may vary depending on each person treated) and if used for extended periods of time. In my opinion, non-steroidal adrenal support supplements are safer and usually all that is needed for most cases of adrenal fatigue.

How does a patient know if they have adrenal fatigue? Blood adrenal hormone levels can be helpful but are like a "snapshot reading" (a one time level) and since cortisol levels go up when you are stressed, such as at a blood draw, this can affect the snapshot blood level.

This is one of many reasons why saliva testing is recommended because you can conveniently obtain several cortisol-level readings over a 24 hour period to establish the adrenal hormone rhythms.

Saliva testing has been researched and found very accurate by reputable medical groups; in fact it is used to monitor hormone levels in medical research, including that done by World Health Organizations. It is also an approved form of testing, by many major health insurance companies, such as Blue Cross/Blue Shield.

Many pharmacies carry the type manufactured by "ZRT Labs, Inc.", which is also an approved blood lab, so you might check with your pharmacy to see if they carry this brand. Most adrenal saliva tests are not terribly expensive and can be diagnostic in detecting adrenal fatigue.

CHAPTER 3:

Balancing Adrenal Fatigue Treatment with Hypothyroid Therapy

Adrenal Fatigue can be a real dilemma for thyroid patients in many ways and my belief is that this is why some doctors like to stay away from it and one of the ways they do this is by denying its existence (certainly not true of all of them).

Medical sources including the thyroid medication manufacturers warn that "untreated adrenal cortical insufficiency" (low cortisol) can be worsened by treating hypothyroidism with hormone replacement therapy, without first correcting it or treating them both simultaneously. What then becomes a question is - how bad does the low cortisol have to be, to present a real problem? Certainly full blown adrenal insufficiency can present with this problem but it only takes common sense to realize that severe adrenal fatigue or adrenal exhaustion can as well (clinically low cortisol regardless of cause).

Less severe adrenal fatigue many times will resolve when hypothyroidism is corrected.

This is because the low functioning thyroid causes everything, including the adrenal glands to operate low in the body (slowed metabolism). When adrenal fatigue in hypothyroid patients isn't severe, it usually corrects on its own when the hypothyroidism is corrected.

Other patients aren't as fortunate and you can find their testimonials often online. They struggle with their adrenal fatigue worsening when they started thyroid hormone medication and continue to struggle with it as they continue their treatment. Some of them also have intermittent adrenal fatigue that is ongoing or chronic and flares easily with stress or physical exertion, even while they are on optimal thyroid hormone therapy. I personally fit into that category and I had a variety of symptoms that worsened with the start of thyroid hormone medication. I feel it's possible that many of the patients who report worsening symptoms for a while after starting thyroid medication for hypothyroidism, may very well be experiencing these adjustment symptoms as both the thyroid and adrenal hormones are trying to correct to normal levels.

Those who seem to never reach a well adjusted state on thyroid hormone should have their adrenal hormones tested in my opinion.

In regard to cortisol steroids (corticosteroids) that replace low cortisol which include the brands "Prednisone" and "Cortef", I agree with those sources that warn if a doctor is not highly skilled in administering these drugs for adrenal fatigue, they can potentially worsen it (adrenal suppression). I am not adding this fact as anti-cortisol treatment propaganda. I am mentioning it because this warning is a logical one in regard to the administering of steroid treatments of any kind! True adrenal insufficiency is easier to treat in one sense because patients need full replacement as a lifelong treatment, while adrenal fatigue sufferers need less than full replacement and usually for short term. It's possible there is a dose of cortical steroid that is safe to treat adrenal fatigue on a permanent basis but medical research has yet to find it, so that it works for a large cross section of people, safely and with no adverse effects or risks.

If safe over-the-counter supplements can be tried first, this is a better way to treat adrenal fatigue in my opinion. A doctor will be needed for corticosteroid treatment as previously mentioned, if it also needs to be administered for severe adrenal fatigue cases at a certain point.

Helpful over-the-counter supplements for adrenal fatigue include the "B" vitamins, especially B-5, B-6 and B-12, vitamin C, licorice root extract (only as label-recommended) and processed adrenal glandular supplements (usually beef/bovine source), using the same precautions as with licorice root.

Some people report improvement while on herbal adrenal support supplements as well, including use of a supplement called "Adreset", made by the Metagenics Company. This company also makes a vitamin supplement for adrenal support called "Cortico-B5 & B6", which also contains magnesium and vitamin C in it. My pharmacist, who works with local doctors, recommended these to me because they are pharmaceutical grade and they have helped with my flares of adrenal fatigue a great deal.

A company that makes a non-hormone adrenal glandular is Vitamin Research Product Company who offers their product called "CortiTrophin".

Their company has Pharmacists and MDs behind research and development of their supplements and is why I believe they are more reputable than some of the other adrenal supplement manufacturers that are out there.

Much of the medical community still has this condition on a back shelf, until it becomes more widely accepted as a real illness.

CHAPTER 4:

Adrenal Fatigue or "Hypocortisolemia"

With Adrenal Fatigue being one of my areas of interest, I watch for updated research in regard to this subject. Many times I will come across medical research articles in regard to this syndrome but it will be referred-to by other names, such as "mild adrenal insufficiency" or simply a "low cortisol state". Some reputable medical entities still do not believe that an Adrenal Fatigue type disorder exists (less that full-blown adrenal insufficiency), including surprisingly, the Mayo Clinic -- a source I highly respect.

With Adrenal Fatigue, as with more severe adrenal adrenal insufficient states, the hormone "Cortisol" is most commonly the one that becomes low or deficient. It is the hormone that manages stress in the body on a daily basis and provides energy for the body, in a cyclic rhythm. In the recent medical research article I will refer to below, it is referred to as "hypocortisolemia" (another term for low cortisol).

It seems as if some in the medical community avoid the term "Adrenal Fatigue", for reasons I have yet to understand. I do believe in the case of some medical people, they feel anything less than true, full-blown adrenal insufficiency, simply does not exist and so anything recognized that is less than this more severe form of adrenal dysfunction, is a pseudo-syndrome (not legitimate) in their opinion. The problem I have with this attitude is the fact that a number of research articles going back more than two decades, recognize mild adrenal dysfunction or sub-clinically low functioning of the adrenal glands. This includes research articles on Chronic Fatigue Syndrome (CFS), Fibromyalgia and Post Traumatic Stress Disorder (PTSD), which have all been proven in a number of medical research studies, to present with low cortisol levels.

There have in fact been trials of treatments for these disorders, using a cortisol replacement drug (hydrocortisone), with some results being favorable and some that were not favorable, which could be a matter of finding the correct therapeutic dose of the drug, that will relieve symptoms without adverse side effects.

In studies of PTSD patients, there have been favorable outcomes using cortisol replacement in controlled studies, to manage the symptoms of this stress disorder. The research article I refer to below, also points this out. I do not believe it is a coincidence that these syndromes that present with low cortisol, including; CFS and PTSD, are also referred to as "stress syndromes". I also believe that Adrenal Fatigue is a low-cortisol, stress-syndrome and strongly associated with these other syndromes.

The medical research article I wish to refer to is titled; "Stress-induced hypocortisolemia diagnosed as psychiatric disorders responsive to hydrocortisone replacement" (U.S./NIH - PubMed Website).

It is an interesting medical research article in that, it points out the fact that severe early life stressors, can result in later life cortisol hormone deficiencies that are mild-to-moderate. The article also points out that this mild adrenal insufficient state they refer-to in the article as; "hypocortisolemia", is often mistaken for psychiatric disorders.

This correlates with the fact that many people who suffer Adrenal Fatigue, attest to the fact that their symptoms were considered to be psychosomatic, before they were thoroughly tested for cortisol levels and found to be deficient.

The research article recommends testing hormone levels, including cortisol, before prescribing psychotropic medications (antidepressants). A major importance of the article as well, is the fact that low cortisol that is not severe enough to be true adrenal insufficiency, is again recognized. Some of us choose to call this sub-clinical hypo-functioning of the adrenal glands; "Adrenal Fatigue". If medical professionals prefer a different term then they should officially name the syndrome, so that more people in the medical community will recognize it, test for it and treat it.

CHAPTER 5:

CFS, Fibromyalgia and Low Cortisol

For more than two decades, researchers studying Chronic Fatigue Syndrome (CFS) and Fibromyalgia Syndrome, have conducted studies in regard to adrenal function in patients with these syndromes and have concluded that patients are found to be experiencing "low adrenal function" as one of the features of these syndromes. This co-existing condition is also called "adrenal fatigue", "adrenal exhaustion" and "low adrenal reserve" as previously mentioned. Reputable medical sources also state that patients with Thyroid Disease are at higher risk than the general population, for also having co-existing CFS and/or Fibromyalgia.

Through testing of a patient's adrenal hormones, it can be determined if that person has low-functioning adrenals. In addition to blood testing, saliva tests are also accurate for testing the "free levels" of the adrenal hormones, the main ones being DHEA and cortisol. A "24 hour urinary cortisol test" can also be done to test adrenal-cortisol levels.

Another major adrenal function blood test is also available, called the "ACTH Stimulation Test". This one is designed to confirm or rule out true "adrenal insufficiency" (full blown). Most CFS and Fibromyalgia patients do not have true, full blown adrenal insufficiency but a milder form of adrenal fatigue/exhaustion.

Conclusions by major medical research groups, including the NIH, state that low cortical levels, are found to be a contributing factor in CFS/FMS, due to dysfunction of the HPA Axis (Hypothalamus-Pituitary-Adrenal Axis). It is my opinion because of this, that CFS/FMS has as one of its features, a form of adrenal fatigue, that does not meet the definition for true "adrenal insufficiency" and because of this, it cannot be medically treated the same. With full blown Adrenal Insufficiency, the low adrenal hormones must be replaced through steroid treatment (cortisone-steroid/hydrocortisone). With lesser forms of low adrenal function, such as adrenal fatigue, steroid treatment can possibly worsen the adrenal problem because the steroids may cause "adrenal suppression". This means the patient may have to take the steroids, the rest of their life because anything less than very short-term use of the steroids, can cause this suppression.

This milder form of low adrenal function, many times is treated with natural supplements (previously listed) such as DHEA, adrenal glandular and multi-vitamins that contain those that help boost adrenal function, as well as B-12 shots. These are all over-the-counter supplements, with the exception of B-12 shots but you can also obtain B-12 in oral form that is over-the-counter. All of these supplements have been found to be helpful in resolving adrenal fatigue conditions.

Some of the other things medical researchers have studied in regard to CFS and Fibromyalgia, is the fact that these syndromes can have different triggers for different patients but with many, it is an underlying viral, autoimmune, bacterial etc…, type infection in the body, that causes chronic activation of the immune system and over time, this uses up some of the adrenal reserves.

The adrenals serve a major role in releasing cortisol, the body's natural anti-inflammatory, attempting to ward off inflammation. Cortisol (also called "cortical"), is also the "stress hormone", that helps the body to deal with stress of all kinds, without it, even the smallest stressor would cause shock and death (adrenal crises).

It, along with adrenaline, are considered to be "fight or flight" hormones as well and help protect the body from the effects of stress, from minor emotional stressors, to major ones, such as a car accident or a serious disease (post traumatic).

This in my opinion is why persons with CFS/FMS have such low tolerance for stressors both emotional and physical. With low adrenal function, even mild emotional and physical stressors result in major fatigue. Couple this with the immune system dysfunction that CFS/FMS patients also experience and you have syndromes with serious symptoms that can greatly impact quality-of-life. It may be that the immune deficiency found in both CFS and Fibromyalgia is also a type of burn-out of that system, due to constant, ongoing activation of it, that the body eventually loses the ability to continue.

As with all other opinions about CFS and Fibromyalgia, we have to consider all of the above, as some of the many theories that are out there however, I feel the evidence of low adrenal function in CFS and Fibromyalgia, is overwhelming. What I have described, is what I feel connects these syndromes to a form of adrenal fatigue.

CHAPTER 6:

Conditions That Cause Mild Adrenal Insufficiency

Adrenal insufficiency is a condition in which the adrenal glands do not produce enough hormones to aid in regulating the body's metabolism, stress coping, controlling inflammation and sexual functioning. The main adrenal hormone that becomes low with this condition is "cortisol" as mentioned in previous chapters and when low levels are detected in a person, it is sometimes referred to as "hypocortisolemia". Full blown adrenal insufficiency is referred to as "Addison's Disease." There are, however, milder forms of adrenal dysfunction as listed below. Some statistics state that about 10% of people with thyroid disease experience a degree of mild adrenal insufficiency.

Post Traumatic Stress Disorder. This condition, abbreviated PTSD, is a traumatic stress-caused condition that is also considered to be an anxiety disorder.

People experience the onset of this disorder as a result of severe traumatizing experiences, such as car accidents, acts of violence that are perpetrated upon them, the sudden loss of a loved one or having been in active combat during wartime. The severe shock caused to the body from such incidents can cause the glands regulating adrenal hormone output to become "blunted", meaning they begin to function at a sub-normal level. While their adrenal hormones may remain within normal limits, they will be at lower or lowest normal (borderline low), which causes them to have an inability to cope with stressors.

Research studies on PTSD that are published by reputable medical groups (including the U.S. National Institutes of Health) state that low cortisol levels found in patients with this disorder, may contribute to their symptoms of anxiety, insomnia and flashbacks, meaning they may mentally relive their traumatic experiences repeatedly. In controlled test studies, using cortisol supplementation to treat PTSD patients, results showed that symptoms were reduced significantly by carefully monitored physiological dosing to increase their low level of the stress hormone.

Chronic Fatigue Syndrome (CFS). This condition has also been found to cause a low level of the stress hormone cortisol evidenced by analyzing the blood and urine cortisol levels in people who experience the illness. Research studies on CFS have repeatedly confirmed this fact and have also found that patients report that they were experiencing chronic or sudden severe stress just before the onset of the illness. This would mean that CFS is very possibly also a stress-related condition that causes the adrenal hormone regulating glands in the body to become blunted.

The U.S. National Institutes of Health released a report in October of 1996, in which they found through a controlled study, that cortisol supplementation/replacement in patients with CFS had a benefit but was found to be short-lived. Afterward, some patients began experiencing a more severe form of adrenal suppression, meaning it caused a worsening of their adrenal insufficiency after a few weeks on the cortisol replacement drug.

Fibromyalga Syndrome (FMS). Being very similar to CFS, Fibromyalgia also has fatigue as a major symptom. The aspect that sets this illness apart from CFS is the widespread body pain that is not found to be as prominent in CFS patients. Despite this fact, researchers studying both illnesses have found them to have 75% crossover similarities. This includes the fact that FMS patients often report chronic stress as being a factor in their development of the illness.

A number of research studies have also found cortisol levels to be low in FMS patients and controlled trials of cortisol supplementation have been conducted to determine if there would be a benefit for these patients. The findings were similar to those found when supplementing CFS patients with cortisol hormone replacement and while some patients improved, the long-term risks for using the drug did not merit establishing it as a medically recognized treatment for FMS.

Adrenal Fatigue. This sub-clinical form of adrenal insufficiency is still not recognized widely by the medical community, although certain types of doctors recognize the disorder.

This includes MDs who practice holistic treatments, Naturopaths and Osteopathic Physicians. With this syndrome which is also referred to as a condition of "low adrenal reserves" and "adrenal exhaustion", many of the symptoms found in CFS and FMS are not present, including joint and muscle pain and other inflammatory problems in the body. Adrenal Fatigue is strictly a condition causing mild to moderate fatigue and reduced stress tolerance. Some medical sources are stating that adrenal fatigue that is prolonged and not treated, through proper rest, improved diet, adrenal boosting natural supplements and reducing contributing stressors, may result in the condition becoming a precursor (a pre-condition) to CFS and FMS.

While the conditions listed above are commonly found to cause mild adrenal insufficiency, other conditions can also be a cause or contributing factor, including other chronic, inflammatory and autoimmune diseases that contribute to increased stress levels in the body. See a professional, licensed physician for a complete evaluation if you suspect that you may be suffering from a health condition causing mild adrenal insufficiency.

CHAPTER 7:

Cortisol & DHEA Supplements for Adrenal Fatigue

Since the year 2004, I have written a lot on the subject of mild hypo-cortisolism that is found in different conditions, that for lack of another well-established term, we call "adrenal fatigue" but it is often during the research I'm doing at any given time for articles etc..., that I often find, that many in the medical community still do not recognize mild forms of adrenal insufficiency and they do not believe that adrenal fatigue syndromes exist.

I actually hope Doctors or medically knowledgeable people of any type, will at some point make a suggestion for a name that doesn't come across as bogus for the syndrome and at the same time, if they don't believe sub-clinical forms of adrenal hypo-cortisolism exist, to also explain why all of the research articles that describe it, are somehow all collectively wrong on the subject (the later challenge will be much more difficult).

The majority of adrenal fatigue patients will at times have snap-shot readings that are normal, when blood tested for cortisol levels.

They will also pass the ACTH Stimulation Test (confirms or rules out full blown adrenal insufficiency) and is why it is recommended to obtain multiple readings throughout the day, via saliva cortisol testing for milder forms of adrenal hypo-cortisolism.

When I personally had the ACTH Stimulation Test performed on me, my cortisol reading was about mid-range on the baseline reading however, I was anxious before and during the test and it's better to obtain cortisol rhythm of multi-readings during a normal activity day. Even though I had a normal baseline on that ACTH Stimulation Test, I also had a 24 hour urinary test through an endocrinologist's office and my cortisol averaged "10.7", with normal range at the lab being <119 for males ages 18 and above. To be in the middle of that range (mid-level), I would have had to register a result of about a 50 or 60 and my Dr. admitted that mine was a very low reading for a 24 hour urine cortisol test. This confirmed that I didn't have true, full-blown adrenal insufficiency but that I did have a serious case of adrenal fatigue.

In medical research studies, in which patients with different diseases, are found to have low cortisol levels, the medical investigators are usually referring to "low cortisol" as being in the low-normal range, so it is low compared to "controls" and low compared to normal subjects. They even give the number differences, calling them "significant" even when the difference is only 2 or 3 points lower than normal subjects have.

One statement the NIH makes in their Centers For Disease Control study of CFS, that has always struck me as important is this one; "Doctors have long known that even subtle deficiencies in cortisol is associated with lethargy and fatigue" (Oct, 1996).

How Does DHEA Supplementation Factor into This?

I've lately come more to the conclusion that I've suspected from the beginning of my search and research on adrenal fatigue, that supplementing with DHEA, will help low DHEA levels but usually doesn't help with low cortisol.

Maybe in some patients it does help to raise cortisol, once the circle of conversion goes completely around but there's conflicting information about DHEA out there. What will help the adrenals to produce more cortisol, are vitamins that support adrenal function, rest and adequate sleep and if needed, the safe and cautious use of licorice extract and adrenal glandular extracts. Some Doctors also sometimes prescribe "pregnenolone" to adrenal fatigue patients or other combinations of hormones to help with the cycle of conversion that occurs between the precursor types (those that convert into sex hormones, including pregnenolone).

A lot of medical resources state that the majority of women can safely take 25mg or less of DHEA and there is very low risk of it causing their androgen levels (male hormones) to go too high and men are supposed to be able to take up to 50mg safely.

I don't feel DHEA would suppress cortisol to a significant degree at these doses but the point is that they also might not help raise cortisol, so that taking it alone, could cause more of a DHEA to cortisol ratio imbalance.

This isn't true of people who have low DHEA but normal cortisol levels, because DHEA is all they need in these cases.

The Journal of Pharmacology has a research article that states that patients with Crohn's Disease and Lupus, are one example of low DHEA, that when supplemented, improves symptoms of these diseases but DHEA can become low for other reasons as well.

In Some Cases Cortisol Supplementation is the Answer

The "American Psychiatric Association", made a statement in the "American Journal of Phychiatry", in a research test that was conducted by 3 psychiatrists and 6 MDs. They stated that supplementing Post Traumatic Stress Disorder patients (PTSD) with low-dose cortisol, can help them due to the fact that the low cortisol, is a major factor in causing symptoms of the illness.

This study, which didn't go overboard with the dosing of cortisol, like other studies have in the past, such as those experimenting with cortisol supplementing in CFS patients, had more favorable results at the lower-dose treatments that were administered.

There are now newer studies reported by the major medical research publishing groups that show that CFS patients did improve with lower-dose cortisol treatment. These studies are more recent than those that reported "adrenal suppression" and other adverse effects at higher dose treatments.

Cortisol replacement therapy is only available by prescription, by a licensed medical professional but hopefully as more research is done, they will find a safe dose that will help treat adrenal fatigue type syndromes.

CHAPTER 8:

The Role Stress in Diseases and Syndromes

Stress is a known trigger for adrenal fatigue and related syndromes, such as Chronic Fatigue Syndrome and Fibromyalgia and can also bring an autoimmune disease to the surface that is in the body but hasn't fully manifested. Thyroid diseases are some of the more common health disorders that can be triggered by stress, especially Grave's Disease/hyperthyroidism.

PTSD (Post Traumatic stress Disorder) is also a chronic stress caused syndrome but is also classified as an anxiety disorder.

I personally went through an extreme period of chronic stress and my thyroid disease, called "Hashimoto's Thyroiditis", manifested as a result as well as a severe case of adrenal fatigue. I was left untreated for these disorders for several months and as a result experienced a severe flare-up in the year 2003 that also triggered the onset of Chronic Fatigue Syndrome, which I continue to struggle with to date.

I initially developed a severe case of hives and a strange viral type illness that left me with the co-occurring CFS. Afterward, the lymph nodes in my neck remained mildly swollen to this day and I also suffer multiple chemical sensitivities (MCS).

My belief is that CFS is a syndrome causing an altered HPA Axis (Hypothalamus-Pituitary-Adrenal glands), plus altered immune system function (deficiency). I suggest to people who suspect they have adrenal fatigue, CFS or a chronic illness/disease to have their adrenal hormones and all other hormones (including the sex ones) checked as well because it is my belief that hormonal imbalances over time, can possibly result in CFS and Fibromyalgia type illnesses.

Some who have read my articles online or my posts on forums, may wonder why I have the passion I do for the adrenal syndrome subjects and it is because it is my belief that adrenal fatigue can eventually cause CFS and/or FMS type syndromes, when not diagnosed and treated as early as possible.

Another strong association to these type syndromes is EBV (Epstein-Barr Virus), which causes mononucleosis initially in some patients but afterward, remains in a persons body for life.

This virus is suspected of having a strong connection to CFS. While most people have EBV in their system beginning in childhood (estimates are 80 to 95% of the population), most only have antibody titers to the virus, that are just barely positive, like a "5", a "10", "20" above normal, etc..., others actually have flare-ups of this virus (reactivation), probably due to a compromised immune system (immune deficiency) that causes high titers of the virus to replicate in their bodies over time.

Many in the medical field are of the opinion that EBV is a background virus like many others in the herpes virus-family that can flare repeatedly like cold sores can (also a herpes virus that remains in the system). When flare-ups happen, they believe it can cause or at least contribute to symptoms of CFS in some people.

In my case, my EBV antibodies count was "218" with normal range being <20 (below 20), so mine was more than ten times the normal cut off range.

Some Doctors believe the EBV test means nothing, unless actually being used to test for active mononucleosis but there has to be a reason some patient's EBV counts elevate so highly.

Both MDs who treat me for hypothyroidism and CFS, believe that EBV can flare/reactivate in some patients who have the higher titers of the virus in their system. Many sources also state that adrenal fatigue is a major feature of this because the adrenal glands are the major moderators of the immune system.

While EBV may not be the actual root cause of CFS, it has been shown to be an indicator of immune dysfunction in studies that have been conducted. In my opinion, it is just one of many factors that can contribute to the symptoms of CFS.

The Centers for Disease Control/U.S. Gov., has been publishing studies and diagnostic criteria for CFS, for many years, so it is recognized as a real illness, regardless of the reluctance on the part of some medical doctors to recognize it.

Many patients with CFS have complete remission of it within two to five years while others have partial but significant improvement, even if it never completely remits. Some may have it for many years but regardless, it does not cause organ damage or decrease life span expectancy, according to published medical research.

It also does not negatively affect intellect; despite the "brain fog" symptoms it also causes in patients who experience it (i.e. difficulty concentrating and short term memory loss).

Things that speed recovery for CFS, are; treating the associated adrenal fatigue, getting proper sleep and rest, a healthy diet, exercising to tolerance and making sure other diseases a patient might have are treated. Under-treatment of a thyroid disorder for example, can serve as a trigger for continuing CFS flare-ups and may actually be a trigger for the syndrome itself according to some medical sources. Many sources also state that thyroid patients commonly have co-occurring CFS and/or Fibromyalgia (these syndromes have 75% crossover symptoms).

CHAPTER 9:

Another Look at Adrenal Fatigue Treatments

There are non-steroidal treatments that can help resolve adrenal fatigue as previously mentioned, including supplements, such as an over-the-counter adrenal hormone called "DHEA", which when taken at the recommended dose, will convert into other needed hormones, including the sex ones. I will add that with DHEA, you need your doctor to help you decide what dose-level is safe for you via testing of your current blood level of the hormone.

There are also "adrenal glandular extracts" that contain animal adrenal glands, usually bovine (beef) that have been reported for many years to help patients regain normal adrenal function. There is also "licorice root extract", that research has found helps patients with adrenal fatigue, to produce higher levels of the stress regulating hormone; "cortisol". An important energy-producing enzyme called "Co-Q10" can also be a beneficial supplement, due to its effects in helping tokeep bodily tissues properly oxygenated.

Multivitamins and minerals can also be very helpful, especially the "B' vitamins (like B-12, B-5 & B-6) and minerals such as magnesium, potassium, and zinc.

Why in the world these things that might be called "natural remedies", are sometimes given a "bad rap", I'll never know! I feel it is ludicrous for anyone, including someone who is a medical professional, to feel something must be a synthetic in order to be effective. This is an incredible view since the vast majority of what keeps us healthy, are nutrients that occur naturally. Let's give God or Nature (if you prefer), the credit for having enough sense to provide us with a few things to keep us healthy and to heal us!

I am not against synthetic medications, they are lifesavers and tremendously effective but when the idea is implied that there is no treatment for a condition, unless it is severe enough to be treated with a synthetic, I will disagree 100%. It is sometimes claimed that pharmaceuticals are the only available treatments, when there are obviously other helpful non-prescription treatments available.

It is a complete and total shame, to allow patients who can benefit from these, to continue suffering rather than giving them a trial of them.

Natural versus Pharmaceutical? – Both should be Options

I'll just make a few more statements, hopefully that point to the fact that there are no perfect answers for many aspects of this debate in regard to "natural versus pharmaceutical" although there is a general guidance we all know to follow that even common sense points out to us.

Licensed medical practitioners obviously are those called to heal and treat people who have illnesses and to keep them well (preventative). The first line of reasoning is to see a doctor when you need medical treatment. Conventional medicine and pharmaceutical drugs have saved lives, extended lives and restored quality of life.

Natural remedies have had miraculously positive and healing effects on some people as well, that conventional treatments failed to resolve. Some natural supplements are far safer than others and just as with pharmaceuticals, they do not have the same effect on each individual.

Some people have been known to have severely adverse effects from naturals (uncommon) and others have actually died from them (very rare and usually due to misuse or abuse of them).

The same is true of some pharmaceuticals. SSRI antidepressant labels for example are now required by the FDA to include mention that some people have become suicidal when taking the drugs, especially younger people. I know for a fact that cases of suicide have occurred in those prescribed the drugs but is a rare occurance. Does this mean SSRI's should be sloughed-off as harmful? Absolutely not, - some people could not survive without them.

On the other hand, naturals cannot be sloughed-off either and in fact, they were placed here by God or nature if you prefer for the very purpose of healing and keeping things well. Pharmaceutical drug-evolution actually came from natural remedies in many cases.

Now, in regard to articles and books/e-books (like this one) on the subject of health treatments, both natural and prescribed; there are simply too many "ins and outs" for any one side of the argument to claim they have the best answers on all aspects.

That's almost like saying there is only one correct or perfect political or religious view on all aspects of those controversial subjects. It is simply not going to happen.

Even in the medical field, certain types of MDs do not see Osteopath doctors as being as legitimate as other types of MDs and others do not recognize naturopaths as being legitimate at all. This despite the fact that they can be legally accredited after required studies to practice with a license in those fields. As far as "quacks" go, and I say this respectfully, there are quacks in every field, including MDs, Natural Remedy people, police officers, ministers, dentists, article/book writers, etc...

Never should this fact cause us to see everyone in light of the bad apples that exist in their fields. Moderation should be done, in all of these fields. MDs have to answer to medical boards, ministers to the clergy of their denomination and article writers, to the websites they write for.

What's my point? Well, I first of all feel it doesn't hurt to have these type discussions in-balance for perspective-sake. I do believe however that there are and never will be perfect answers for every aspect of this subject.

I wish there were always definitive answers but this is simply not true in many cases. That's life and the world we live in and also why we have to maintain our individuality and make thoughtful decisions the best we can and then pray (or hope) for the best outcomes.

My Own Positive Experiences with Natural Supplements

I have mentioned previously, my positive experiences with supplements that help significantly when I experience flares of adrenal fatigue. I have seen benefits with naturals among my family members as well. My wife suffered severe yeast infections for 15 years that were intermittent but caused lots of agony when they did occur. She went to several doctors and each recommended prescriptions, some that helped temporarily. One of the last doctors she went-to prescribed a dangerous regimen of Diflucan (ten 200mg pills taken for 10 days). The reason she did not have the prescription filled is because the pharmacist's jaw almost fell to the floor when he saw the prescription and told her if she took the highest dose for 10 days, irreversible liver and/or kidney damage could potentially occur.

Someone had been recommending she take probiotics and acidophilus (natural supplements) and she finally took the advice and upon taking a regimen of these two natural supplements, she complete recovery from the yeast infections. She was absolutely thrilled.

Even this example is not to say every person would see the same results but this made us realized naturals cannot be dismissed. Some things in the natural category are absolutely needed, which includes Vitamin B12 that if some people did not take, would cause them to die from pernicious anemia. The same is true with people who need iron for other types of anemia and calcium supplementation due to parathyroid imbalance etc... Pharmaceuticals can have the same life-saving, sustaining and healing benefits so I feel doctors should be willing to see a balance between the two in cases when either or both can benefit.

Determining when, a conventional treatment is better than a natural treatment and vise versa, can be a difficult subject with lots of details and factors involved.

Some issues involving the conventional versus natural treatments debate include disagreements about when they should be combined or when one is a better option than the other, etc.... and it really becomes complicated at times. Patients are often caught in the middle not knowing which direction to turn. Those suffering severe symptoms from health disorders and diseases as I have suffered myself at times, are very willing to look at every possible legitimate avenue to find relief. In short, there are not always simple answers although we all wish the way was unmistakably clear in every case.

One thing I have always made sure of is to mention in each article or book/e-book I've written that includes reference to natural supplements (non-prescription, over-the-counter), that patients run them past their doctors for approval, before taking them. I've always done this going back six years to my beginnings in writing on health subjects because I know that all treatments don't have the same effect on each and every person.

I mention in a recent article I wrote, a test a person can do at home using one drop of iodine on the soft area of their arm and observing the spot it makes to see if the iodine absorbs quickly or slowly. When quickly absorbed, this possibly indicates the thyroid is starving for iodine or is in need of more due to inadequate thyroid hormone production. I gave a lot of thought to adding this self-test into the article I was writing because there are doctors out there who disagree that the iodine spot test has any legitimacy whatsoever. I also mention several times in the article that tests like these cannot diagnose and that only qualified doctors can diagnose thyroid disorders.

The reason I added mention of this test into the article however was for several reasons, one of which I will now describe:

I called-in live, to a health T.V. show, on which Dr. Sherri Tenpenny was a guest, back in about the year 2003 or 2004 (still have the show on tape) and told her I had three abnormal readings on some thyroid lab tests, that were done due to symptoms of an under active thyroid I was having but that my doctor at the time was delaying treatment because my TSH was not reaching "10.0 or higher" (pituitary hormone that elevates with hypothyroidism).

It in fact it was at "8.3" (my T3 uptake was also flagged low) but she mentioned that if my case was caused by Hashimoto's thyroiditis, there could also be antibodies blocking thyroid hormones. She suggested I do an in-home iodine spot test using "Lugol's solution" (iodine product).

I bought a bottle of the iodine and had my non-thyroid diseased family members to also place iodine drops on their inside upper arm areas at the same time I did. Their spots stayed for an entire day, while mine absorbed within one-hour. I waited a few days and did the test again with same results (very fast absorption). I then had blood testing for thyroid antibodies a few months later (immune cells that cause disease) and Hashimoto's thyroiditis was revealed, my anti-TG ABs coming in at "537" with normal range being "<35". Both my TPO and TG ABs are highly elevated when re-rested each year but I am at least now treated for my thyroid disorder. I was amazed that Dr. Tenpenny accurately predicted my case as being autoimmune thyroiditis.

Dr. Tenpenny is Board Certified in emergency medicine and is an osteopath doctor and very well-known and recognized as an expert in many areas, including vaccinations.

Natural and Prescribed Treatments for Adrenal Fatigue

These type MDs can not only be board certified but can perform surgeries, deliver babies etc.... . I found however that some MDs in other fields look at osteopaths almost in the same category as naturopaths when they are in-fact qualified in far more areas of practice. My point being that there are qualified doctors in both the conventional and natural medical fields and many practice aspects of both.

53

CHAPTER 10:

The Importance in Confirming Treatment Information

Some non-pro medical subject authors (like me) do a good job in relating information about available treatments because they have thoroughly researched. I also agree that articles on medical subjects should be backed by information that can be confirmed but for perspective and balance on this issue and by no means wanting to come across offensive, let me add the following.

One of the major reasons non medical professionals have resorted to search, research and writing medical-subject articles, is due to their not being reasonably informed about their medical conditions by their doctors. Doctors are overbooked and overworked and they simply do not have the time to educate patients beyond the very basic things. Some readers at this point of this chapter might ask "Why would a patient need to know details of their health disorders anyway?" The answer is, first of all because they have a right to know. The illnesses they experience in many cases are life-altering, possibly debilitating and lifelong.

Secondly, doctors can give incorrect diagnoses and whether everyone who may consider this aspect wants to believe it or not, patients many times find corrected diagnoses because they become self-educated enough to spot a wrong diagnosis.

Giving myself for example, I am an autoimmune thyroid disease patient who was diagnosed with hypothyroidism in 2003 but I first experienced a period of hyperthyroidism (overactive thyroid gland). The first two doctors I went to, resorted to snap diagnoses and prescribed antidepressants, claiming my problems were emotional. Strangely, many of my symptoms didn't match those of anxiety and/or depression even though I stated them clearly (i.e. very dry skin, sudden rapid weight loss with no change in diet, hair breaking off, muscle weakness etc.......). I finally literally had to demand blood testing and the thyroid disease was revealed immediately, including highly elevated auto-antibody levels.

After diagnosis, I was under-treated for two years by doctors who did not know how to properly administer thyroid hormone replacement therapy. How do I know this?

Because an Endocrinologist I finally made an appointment with was appalled at the bad treatment I was receiving, once reviewing my medical records.

These type things are why I began search and research extensively. Let me add that I've had doctors tell me I was incorrect about something I researched on very reputable medical sources and upon inquiring with other doctors, found that the initial doctor was incorrect on some very important things.

In regard to my health articles, I can say with absoluteness that anything found in them can be confirmed. I in fact will not include anything in one that can't be confirmed by numerous reputable, reliable sources (medical ones). On very rare occasions I will mention speculation and will state it as such, also mentioning that medical research has yet to find the definitive answer.

Just to add one more example in this area, I'll refer to another thyroid patient advocate and fellow adrenal fatigue sufferer named Mary Shomon, who is also not a medical professional but a very professional writer of medical subjects.

Her story is very similar to mine, in that she was forced to research due to difficulty getting doctors to order proper blood testing and afterward difficulty in receiving proper treatment for her hypothyroidism. Since I began my own self-educating, I have corresponded with 1,000s of patients (not an exaggeration) and have heard my story reflected back to me in their similar experiences. Most were offered antidepressants as I was before diagnostic testing revealed what treatment was actually needed. They would not have even known what to ask for had they not become proactive and self-educated.

I realize I did not start this part of the chapter talking about medical doctors per se but about "medical writers", however, most write for the benefit of other medical professionals. It is almost as if patients are not given the benefit of the doubt for having some intelligence of their own and as if some medical people literally try to withhold information from patients. They are in-essence saying "Put your complete trust in us and don't ask questions and don't double check us (confirm)." If some patients did not do this however, they would not have received treatments that sometimes were lifesaving.

This is not meant as disrespect but there are medical practitioners who fall short. This is why people resort to second opinions. There are also fantastic doctors out there (the majority) but without at least some education on the part of patients, they might not know whether a doctor is good or is one who is about to let them go down hill very fast health-wise.

By no-means was this meant to degrade the medical profession (Thank God for them!) but I felt it very important to explain why in my case, I began to share needed information with fellow-patients. Money had absolutely nothing to do with it and I wrote online for two years not seeking compensation of any kind. I had and do have genuine compassion for others who are going through what I went through before being properly treated for their thyroid disease and adrenal fatigue.

I believe health articles written by non-medical professionals should be confirmed within reason, as long as motives for doing so are always genuine and not an attempt toward censorship. The vast majority of online medical-subject articles are by non-medical professionals as it is and I'm sure there are unreliable ones out there.

I also believe there are some medical ones, written by professionals that contain unreliable information as well. Some of the medical fields have strong disagreements with each other as well, such as conventional MDs who do not agree with holistic approaches used by some Osteopath doctors, etc...

You can see from this and other of my articles that this is an area of heart for me. The bottom line is that some patients are in desperate need of information and sometimes need to hear from fellow-patients they can relate-to.

Finally in closing this book -- my suggestion to thyroid patients, who begin thyroid hormone replacement medication and have a negative reaction to it, is to ask for tests of their adrenal hormone levels.

Not only can your Doctor order blood tests of your adrenal hormone levels but there are also home "saliva tests", that are available via, online mail order and through Pharmacies that medical research has concluded are as accurate for testing the "free levels" of circulating adrenal hormones as serum blood tests are.

One company that offers adrenal saliva test kits online and through many pharmacies nationwide is "ZRT Labs, Inc." founded by biochemist and breast cancer researcher, David T. Zava, (PhD).

Confirming the existence of adrenal fatigue is the first important step toward getting proper treatment for symptoms and to possibly see complete recovery from this common but serious stress related syndrome.

(END)